My Pregnancy Journal

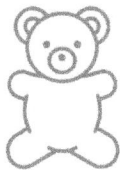

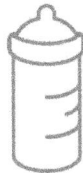

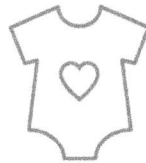

THIS BOOK BELONGS TO

_____

_____

_____

Dedication

This Pregnancy Journal is dedicated to all the wonderful new moms who want to capture key moments of their pregnancy.

You are my inspiration for producing this book and I'm honored to be a part of your experience-from bump to baby.

How to Use this Book

This Pregnancy Journal book will help guide you throughout your pregnancy: prenatal, self care, meal trackers, appointments and more.

Here are examples of daily tracking, checklists and prompts for you to fill in and write about your experience:

1. Finding out- your experience on finding out the big news

2. Birth Plan- fill out information about your plans

3. Baby Name Ideas- write ideas for baby names

4. Appointment Tracker- keep track of all your appointments

5. Weight Log- fill in weekly

6. Prenatal Visits- record key information about your visits

7. Trimester Notes- create checklists for each trimester

8. Meal Planner- fill in daily meals for breakfast, lunch, dinner and snacks

9. Baby to Bump- fill in weekly notes for symptoms, thoughts and feelings, notes to baby, belly photo and more

Finding Out

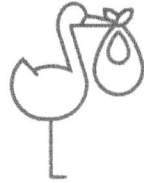

DUE DATE:	

HOW I FOUND OUT:	
WHEN I FOUND OUT:	
MY REACTION:	
HUBBY'S REACTION:	
PARENT'S REACTION:	

WHAT I AM EXCITED ABOUT

WHO I TOLD FIRST

WHAT I WANT YOU TO KNOW

Birth Plan

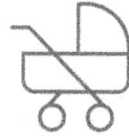

mother's information

NAME:

DUE DATE:

ADDRESS:

O.B.

CONTACT PERSON:

PHONE NUMBER:

LABOR:

I WOULD LIKE TO BE OFFERED AN EPIDURAL	O YES	O NO
I WOULD LIKE TO LABOR IN THE TUB OR SHOWER	O YES	O NO
PLEASE LIMIT CERVICAL CHECKS	O YES	O NO
I WOULD LIKE MY WATER TO BREAK ON ITS OWN	O YES	O NO

DELIVERY:

I WOULD LIKE TO CHOOSE THE POSITION I PUSH IN	O YES	O NO
I WOULD LIKE TO BE COACHED ON HOW TO PUSH	O YES	O NO
I WOULD LIKE TO USE A MIRROR DURING PUSHING	O YES	O NO
I WOULD PREFER TO TEAR NATURALLY VS. AN EPISIOTOMY	O YES	O NO
I'D PREFER A VACUUM DELIVERY OVER FORCEPS	O YES	O NO

Baby Name Ideas

BOY FIRST NAMES	GIRL FIRST NAMES

BOY MIDDLE NAMES	GIRL MIDDLE NAMES

Hospital Bag Checklist

FOR MOMMY

O PAJAMAS

O SOCKS

O SLIPPERS / FLIP FLOPS

O SWEATER

O MATERNITY CLOTHES

O NURSING BRAS

O UNDERWEAR

O TOOTHBRUSH

O TOOTH PASTE

O SHOWER ESSENTIALS

O HAIR TIES / HEADBAND

O HAIR BRUSH

FOR BABY

O RECEIVING BLANKETS

O BABY SOCKS

O BABY MITTENS / HAT

O ONESIES / SLEEPERS

O GOING HOME OUTFIT

O DIAPERS

O BABY WIPES

IMPORTANT

O INSURANCE INFORMATION

O BIRTH PLAN

O DRIVER'S LICENSE

O OB CONTACT INFORMATION

O PEDIATRICIAN CONTACT
INFORMATION

O SOCIAL SECURITY CARD

Appointment Tracker

DATE	DOCTOR	NOTES

Appointment Tracker

DATE	DOCTOR	NOTES

Appointment Tracker

DATE	DOCTOR	NOTES

Weight Log

WEEK #	WEIGHT (LBS.)	WEEK #	WEIGHT (LBS.)
1		21	
2		22	
3		23	
4		24	
5		25	
6		26	
7		27	
8		28	
9		29	
10		30	
11		31	
12		32	
13		33	
14		34	
15		35	
16		36	
17		37	
18		38	
19		39	
20			

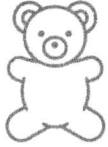

Prenatal Visits

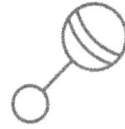

DATE:		SUMMARY OF APPOINTMENT:
WEIGHT:		
BLOOD PRESSURE:		
FETAL HEART RATE:		
DOCTOR:		
NOTES:		
NEXT APPOINTMENT:		

DATE:		SUMMARY OF APPOINTMENT:
WEIGHT:		
BLOOD PRESSURE:		
FETAL HEART RATE:		
DOCTOR:		
NOTES:		
NEXT APPOINTMENT:		

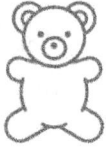

Prenatal Visits

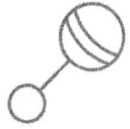

DATE:		SUMMARY OF APPOINTMENT:
WEIGHT:		
BLOOD PRESSURE:		
FETAL HEART RATE:		
DOCTOR:		
NOTES:		
NEXT APPOINTMENT:		

DATE:		SUMMARY OF APPOINTMENT:
WEIGHT:		
BLOOD PRESSURE:		
FETAL HEART RATE:		
DOCTOR:		
NOTES:		
NEXT APPOINTMENT:		

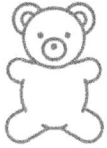

Prenatal Visits

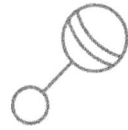

DATE:		SUMMARY OF APPOINTMENT:
WEIGHT:		
BLOOD PRESSURE:		
FETAL HEART RATE:		
DOCTOR:		
NOTES:		
NEXT APPOINTMENT:		

DATE:		SUMMARY OF APPOINTMENT:
WEIGHT:		
BLOOD PRESSURE:		
FETAL HEART RATE:		
DOCTOR:		
NOTES:		
NEXT APPOINTMENT:		

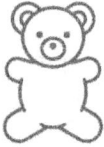

Prenatal Visits

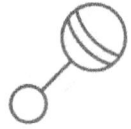

DATE:		SUMMARY OF APPOINTMENT:
WEIGHT:		
BLOOD PRESSURE:		
FETAL HEART RATE:		
DOCTOR:		
NOTES:		
NEXT APPOINTMENT:		

DATE:		SUMMARY OF APPOINTMENT:
WEIGHT:		
BLOOD PRESSURE:		
FETAL HEART RATE:		
DOCTOR:		
NOTES:		
NEXT APPOINTMENT:		

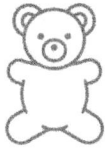

Prenatal Visits

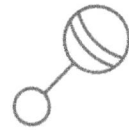

DATE:		SUMMARY OF APPOINTMENT:
WEIGHT:		
BLOOD PRESSURE:		
FETAL HEART RATE:		
DOCTOR:		
NOTES:		
NEXT APPOINTMENT:		

DATE:		SUMMARY OF APPOINTMENT:
WEIGHT:		
BLOOD PRESSURE:		
FETAL HEART RATE:		
DOCTOR:		
NOTES:		
NEXT APPOINTMENT:		

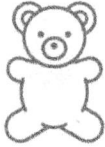

Prenatal Visits

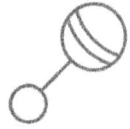

DATE:		SUMMARY OF APPOINTMENT:
WEIGHT:		
BLOOD PRESSURE:		
FETAL HEART RATE:		
DOCTOR:		
NOTES:		
NEXT APPOINTMENT:		

DATE:		SUMMARY OF APPOINTMENT:
WEIGHT:		
BLOOD PRESSURE:		
FETAL HEART RATE:		
DOCTOR:		
NOTES:		
NEXT APPOINTMENT:		

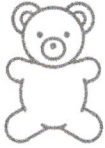

Prenatal Visits

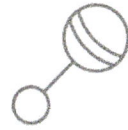

DATE:		SUMMARY OF APPOINTMENT:
WEIGHT:		
BLOOD PRESSURE:		
FETAL HEART RATE:		
DOCTOR:		
NOTES:		
NEXT APPOINTMENT:		

DATE:		SUMMARY OF APPOINTMENT:
WEIGHT:		
BLOOD PRESSURE:		
FETAL HEART RATE:		
DOCTOR:		
NOTES:		
NEXT APPOINTMENT:		

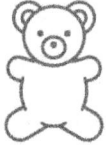

Prenatal Visits

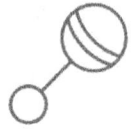

DATE:		SUMMARY OF APPOINTMENT:
WEIGHT:		
BLOOD PRESSURE:		
FETAL HEART RATE:		
DOCTOR:		
NOTES:		
NEXT APPOINTMENT:		

DATE:		SUMMARY OF APPOINTMENT:
WEIGHT:		
BLOOD PRESSURE:		
FETAL HEART RATE:		
DOCTOR:		
NOTES:		
NEXT APPOINTMENT:		

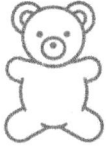

Prenatal Visits

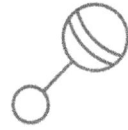

DATE:		SUMMARY OF APPOINTMENT:
WEIGHT:		
BLOOD PRESSURE:		
FETAL HEART RATE:		
DOCTOR:		
NOTES:		
NEXT APPOINTMENT:		

DATE:		SUMMARY OF APPOINTMENT:
WEIGHT:		
BLOOD PRESSURE:		
FETAL HEART RATE:		
DOCTOR:		
NOTES:		
NEXT APPOINTMENT:		

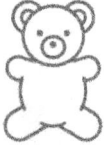

Prenatal Visits

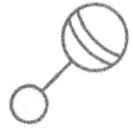

DATE:		SUMMARY OF APPOINTMENT:
WEIGHT:		
BLOOD PRESSURE:		
FETAL HEART RATE:		
DOCTOR:		
NOTES:		
NEXT APPOINTMENT:		

DATE:		SUMMARY OF APPOINTMENT:
WEIGHT:		
BLOOD PRESSURE:		
FETAL HEART RATE:		
DOCTOR:		
NOTES:		
NEXT APPOINTMENT:		

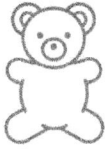

Prenatal Visits

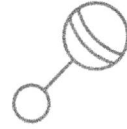

DATE:		SUMMARY OF APPOINTMENT:
WEIGHT:		
BLOOD PRESSURE:		
FETAL HEART RATE:		
DOCTOR:		
NOTES:		
NEXT APPOINTMENT:		

DATE:		SUMMARY OF APPOINTMENT:
WEIGHT:		
BLOOD PRESSURE:		
FETAL HEART RATE:		
DOCTOR:		
NOTES:		
NEXT APPOINTMENT:		

First Trimester

TO DO LIST:

- O
- O
- O
- O
- O
- O
- O
- O
- O
- O
- O
- O
- O
- O
- O
- O
- O
- O
- O
- O
- O
- O
- O
- O

Second Trimester

TO DO LIST:

- O
- O
- O
- O
- O
- O
- O
- O
- O
- O
- O
- O
- O
- O
- O
- O
- O
- O
- O
- O
- O
- O
- O
- O

Third Trimester

TO DO LIST:

- ○
- ○
- ○
- ○
- ○
- ○
- ○
- ○
- ○
- ○
- ○
- ○
- ○
- ○
- ○
- ○
- ○
- ○
- ○
- ○
- ○
- ○

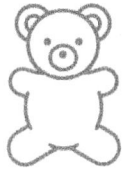

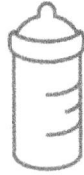

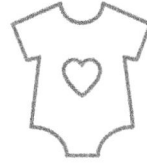

Off To A Great Start

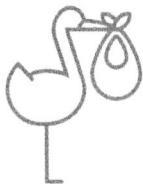

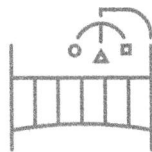

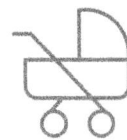

Meal Planner

week number: [　　　　　]   TRIMESTER: O FIRST   O SECOND   O THIRD

	BREAKFAST	LUNCH	DINNER	SNACKS
MONDAY				
	PRENATAL VITAMINS:		WATER:	CUPS
TUESDAY				
	PRENATAL VITAMINS:		WATER:	CUPS
WEDNESDAY				
	PRENATAL VITAMINS:		WATER:	CUPS
THURSDAY				
	PRENATAL VITAMINS:		WATER:	CUPS
FRIDAY				
	PRENATAL VITAMINS:		WATER:	CUPS
SATURDAY				
	PRENATAL VITAMINS:		WATER:	CUPS
SUNDAY				
	PRENATAL VITAMINS:		WATER:	CUPS

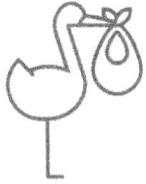

Bump to Baby

week number:

WEIGHT	BELLY SIZE:	DATE

SYMPTOMS:	CRAVINGS AND AVERSIONS:

THOUGHTS AND FEELINGS	BELLY SHOT

NOTES TO BABY:

DEAR BABY,

Meal Planner

week number: [＿＿＿＿＿＿＿] TRIMESTER: O FIRST O SECOND O THIRD

	BREAKFAST	LUNCH	DINNER	SNACKS
MONDAY				
	PRENATAL VITAMINS:		WATER:	CUPS
TUESDAY				
	PRENATAL VITAMINS:		WATER:	CUPS
WEDNESDAY				
	PRENATAL VITAMINS:		WATER:	CUPS
THURSDAY				
	PRENATAL VITAMINS:		WATER:	CUPS
FRIDAY				
	PRENATAL VITAMINS:		WATER:	CUPS
SATURDAY				
	PRENATAL VITAMINS:		WATER:	CUPS
SUNDAY				
	PRENATAL VITAMINS:		WATER:	CUPS

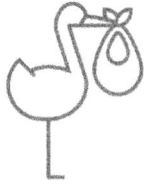

Bump to Baby

week number:

WEIGHT	BELLY SIZE:	DATE

SYMPTOMS:	CRAVINGS AND AVERSIONS:

THOUGHTS AND FEELINGS	BELLY SHOT

NOTES TO BABY:
DEAR BABY,

Meal Planner

week number: [　　　　　　　]　　TRIMESTER:　O FIRST　O SECOND　O THIRD

	BREAKFAST	LUNCH	DINNER	SNACKS
MONDAY				
	PRENATAL VITAMINS:		WATER:	CUPS
TUESDAY				
	PRENATAL VITAMINS:		WATER:	CUPS
WEDNESDAY				
	PRENATAL VITAMINS:		WATER:	CUPS
THURSDAY				
	PRENATAL VITAMINS:		WATER:	CUPS
FRIDAY				
	PRENATAL VITAMINS:		WATER:	CUPS
SATURDAY				
	PRENATAL VITAMINS:		WATER:	CUPS
SUNDAY				
	PRENATAL VITAMINS:		WATER:	CUPS

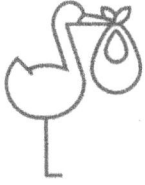

Bump to Baby

week number:

WEIGHT	BELLY SIZE:	DATE

SYMPTOMS:	CRAVINGS AND AVERSIONS:

THOUGHTS AND FEELINGS	BELLY SHOT

NOTES TO BABY:

DEAR BABY,

Meal Planner

week number: [   ] TRIMESTER: O FIRST   O SECOND   O THIRD

	BREAKFAST	LUNCH	DINNER	SNACKS
MONDAY				
	PRENATAL VITAMINS:		WATER:	CUPS
TUESDAY				
	PRENATAL VITAMINS:		WATER:	CUPS
WEDNESDAY				
	PRENATAL VITAMINS:		WATER:	CUPS
THURSDAY				
	PRENATAL VITAMINS:		WATER:	CUPS
FRIDAY				
	PRENATAL VITAMINS:		WATER:	CUPS
SATURDAY				
	PRENATAL VITAMINS:		WATER:	CUPS
SUNDAY				
	PRENATAL VITAMINS:		WATER:	CUPS

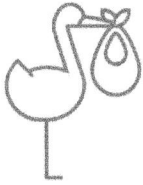

Bump to Baby

week number:

WEIGHT	BELLY SIZE:	DATE

SYMPTOMS:	CRAVINGS AND AVERSIONS:

THOUGHTS AND FEELINGS	BELLY SHOT

NOTES TO BABY:
DEAR BABY,

Meal Planner

week number: [ ] TRIMESTER: O FIRST O SECOND O THIRD

	BREAKFAST	LUNCH	DINNER	SNACKS
MONDAY				
	PRENATAL VITAMINS:		WATER:	CUPS
TUESDAY				
	PRENATAL VITAMINS:		WATER:	CUPS
WEDNESDAY				
	PRENATAL VITAMINS:		WATER:	CUPS
THURSDAY				
	PRENATAL VITAMINS:		WATER:	CUPS
FRIDAY				
	PRENATAL VITAMINS:		WATER:	CUPS
SATURDAY				
	PRENATAL VITAMINS:		WATER:	CUPS
SUNDAY				
	PRENATAL VITAMINS:		WATER:	CUPS

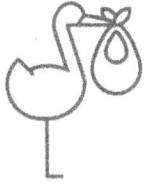

Bump to Baby

week number:

WEIGHT	BELLY SIZE:	DATE

SYMPTOMS:

CRAVINGS AND AVERSIONS:

THOUGHTS AND FEELINGS

BELLY SHOT

NOTES TO BABY:

DEAR BABY,

Meal Planner

week number: [　　　　　　　]　　TRIMESTER:　O FIRST　O SECOND　O THIRD

	BREAKFAST	LUNCH	DINNER	SNACKS
MONDAY				
	PRENATAL VITAMINS:		WATER:	CUPS
TUESDAY				
	PRENATAL VITAMINS:		WATER:	CUPS
WEDNESDAY				
	PRENATAL VITAMINS:		WATER:	CUPS
THURSDAY				
	PRENATAL VITAMINS:		WATER:	CUPS
FRIDAY				
	PRENATAL VITAMINS:		WATER:	CUPS
SATURDAY				
	PRENATAL VITAMINS:		WATER:	CUPS
SUNDAY				
	PRENATAL VITAMINS:		WATER:	CUPS

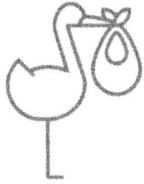

Bump to Baby

week number:

WEIGHT	BELLY SIZE:	DATE

SYMPTOMS:	CRAVINGS AND AVERSIONS:

THOUGHTS AND FEELINGS	BELLY SHOT

NOTES TO BABY:
DEAR BABY,

Meal Planner

week number: [   ]   TRIMESTER: O FIRST   O SECOND   O THIRD

	BREAKFAST	LUNCH	DINNER	SNACKS
MONDAY				
	PRENATAL VITAMINS:		WATER:	CUPS
TUESDAY				
	PRENATAL VITAMINS:		WATER:	CUPS
WEDNESDAY				
	PRENATAL VITAMINS:		WATER:	CUPS
THURSDAY				
	PRENATAL VITAMINS:		WATER:	CUPS
FRIDAY				
	PRENATAL VITAMINS:		WATER:	CUPS
SATURDAY				
	PRENATAL VITAMINS:		WATER:	CUPS
SUNDAY				
	PRENATAL VITAMINS:		WATER:	CUPS

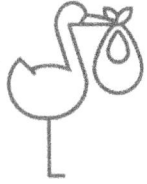

Bump to Baby

week number:

WEIGHT	BELLY SIZE:	DATE

SYMPTOMS:

CRAVINGS AND AVERSIONS:

THOUGHTS AND FEELINGS

BELLY SHOT

NOTES TO BABY:

DEAR BABY,

Meal Planner

week number: [   ]   TRIMESTER: O FIRST   O SECOND   O THIRD

	BREAKFAST	LUNCH	DINNER	SNACKS
MONDAY				
	PRENATAL VITAMINS:		WATER:	CUPS
TUESDAY				
	PRENATAL VITAMINS:		WATER:	CUPS
WEDNESDAY				
	PRENATAL VITAMINS:		WATER:	CUPS
THURSDAY				
	PRENATAL VITAMINS:		WATER:	CUPS
FRIDAY				
	PRENATAL VITAMINS:		WATER:	CUPS
SATURDAY				
	PRENATAL VITAMINS:		WATER:	CUPS
SUNDAY				
	PRENATAL VITAMINS:		WATER:	CUPS

Bump to Baby

week number:

WEIGHT	BELLY SIZE:	DATE

SYMPTOMS:	CRAVINGS AND AVERSIONS:

THOUGHTS AND FEELINGS	BELLY SHOT

NOTES TO BABY:

DEAR BABY,

Meal Planner

week number: [＿＿＿＿＿＿]   TRIMESTER: O FIRST   O SECOND   O THIRD

	BREAKFAST	LUNCH	DINNER	SNACKS
MONDAY				
	PRENATAL VITAMINS:		WATER:	CUPS
TUESDAY				
	PRENATAL VITAMINS:		WATER:	CUPS
WEDNESDAY				
	PRENATAL VITAMINS:		WATER:	CUPS
THURSDAY				
	PRENATAL VITAMINS:		WATER:	CUPS
FRIDAY				
	PRENATAL VITAMINS:		WATER:	CUPS
SATURDAY				
	PRENATAL VITAMINS:		WATER:	CUPS
SUNDAY				
	PRENATAL VITAMINS:		WATER:	CUPS

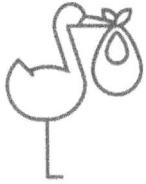

Bump to Baby

week number:

WEIGHT	BELLY SIZE:	DATE

SYMPTOMS:	CRAVINGS AND AVERSIONS:

THOUGHTS AND FEELINGS	BELLY SHOT

NOTES TO BABY:

DEAR BABY,

Meal Planner

week number: [   ]   TRIMESTER: O FIRST   O SECOND   O THIRD

	BREAKFAST	LUNCH	DINNER	SNACKS
MONDAY				
	PRENATAL VITAMINS:		WATER:	CUPS
TUESDAY				
	PRENATAL VITAMINS:		WATER:	CUPS
WEDNESDAY				
	PRENATAL VITAMINS:		WATER:	CUPS
THURSDAY				
	PRENATAL VITAMINS:		WATER:	CUPS
FRIDAY				
	PRENATAL VITAMINS:		WATER:	CUPS
SATURDAY				
	PRENATAL VITAMINS:		WATER:	CUPS
SUNDAY				
	PRENATAL VITAMINS:		WATER:	CUPS

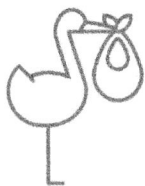

Bump to Baby

week number:

WEIGHT	BELLY SIZE:	DATE

SYMPTOMS:	CRAVINGS AND AVERSIONS:

THOUGHTS AND FEELINGS	BELLY SHOT

NOTES TO BABY:

DEAR BABY,

Meal Planner

week number: [＿＿＿＿＿＿]   TRIMESTER: O FIRST   O SECOND   O THIRD

	BREAKFAST	LUNCH	DINNER	SNACKS
MONDAY				
	PRENATAL VITAMINS:		WATER:	CUPS
TUESDAY				
	PRENATAL VITAMINS:		WATER:	CUPS
WEDNESDAY				
	PRENATAL VITAMINS:		WATER:	CUPS
THURSDAY				
	PRENATAL VITAMINS:		WATER:	CUPS
FRIDAY				
	PRENATAL VITAMINS:		WATER:	CUPS
SATURDAY				
	PRENATAL VITAMINS:		WATER:	CUPS
SUNDAY				
	PRENATAL VITAMINS:		WATER:	CUPS

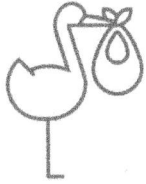

Bump to Baby

week number:

WEIGHT	BELLY SIZE:	DATE

SYMPTOMS:

CRAVINGS AND AVERSIONS:

THOUGHTS AND FEELINGS

BELLY SHOT

NOTES TO BABY:

DEAR BABY,

Meal Planner

week number: [   ]   TRIMESTER: O FIRST   O SECOND   O THIRD

	BREAKFAST	LUNCH	DINNER	SNACKS
MONDAY				
	PRENATAL VITAMINS:		WATER:	CUPS
TUESDAY				
	PRENATAL VITAMINS:		WATER:	CUPS
WEDNESDAY				
	PRENATAL VITAMINS:		WATER:	CUPS
THURSDAY				
	PRENATAL VITAMINS:		WATER:	CUPS
FRIDAY				
	PRENATAL VITAMINS:		WATER:	CUPS
SATURDAY				
	PRENATAL VITAMINS:		WATER:	CUPS
SUNDAY				
	PRENATAL VITAMINS:		WATER:	CUPS

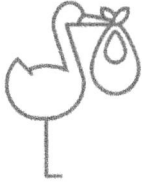

Bump to Baby

week number:

WEIGHT	BELLY SIZE:	DATE

SYMPTOMS:	CRAVINGS AND AVERSIONS:

THOUGHTS AND FEELINGS	BELLY SHOT

NOTES TO BABY:

DEAR BABY,

Meal Planner

week number: [   ]   TRIMESTER: O FIRST   O SECOND   O THIRD

	BREAKFAST	LUNCH	DINNER	SNACKS
MONDAY				
	PRENATAL VITAMINS:		WATER:	CUPS
TUESDAY				
	PRENATAL VITAMINS:		WATER:	CUPS
WEDNESDAY				
	PRENATAL VITAMINS:		WATER:	CUPS
THURSDAY				
	PRENATAL VITAMINS:		WATER:	CUPS
FRIDAY				
	PRENATAL VITAMINS:		WATER:	CUPS
SATURDAY				
	PRENATAL VITAMINS:		WATER:	CUPS
SUNDAY				
	PRENATAL VITAMINS:		WATER:	CUPS

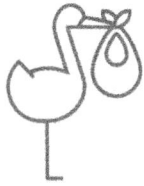

Bump to Baby

week number:

WEIGHT	BELLY SIZE:	DATE

SYMPTOMS:

CRAVINGS AND AVERSIONS:

THOUGHTS AND FEELINGS

BELLY SHOT

NOTES TO BABY:

DEAR BABY,

Meal Planner

week number: [_____]   TRIMESTER: O FIRST   O SECOND   O THIRD

	BREAKFAST	LUNCH	DINNER	SNACKS
MONDAY				
	PRENATAL VITAMINS:		WATER:	CUPS
TUESDAY				
	PRENATAL VITAMINS:		WATER:	CUPS
WEDNESDAY				
	PRENATAL VITAMINS:		WATER:	CUPS
THURSDAY				
	PRENATAL VITAMINS:		WATER:	CUPS
FRIDAY				
	PRENATAL VITAMINS:		WATER:	CUPS
SATURDAY				
	PRENATAL VITAMINS:		WATER:	CUPS
SUNDAY				
	PRENATAL VITAMINS:		WATER:	CUPS

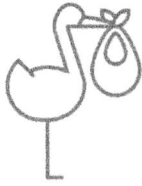

Bump to Baby

week number:

WEIGHT	BELLY SIZE:	DATE

SYMPTOMS:

CRAVINGS AND AVERSIONS:

THOUGHTS AND FEELINGS

BELLY SHOT

NOTES TO BABY:

DEAR BABY,

Meal Planner

week number: [　　　　　　] TRIMESTER: O FIRST O SECOND O THIRD

	BREAKFAST	LUNCH	DINNER	SNACKS
MONDAY				
	PRENATAL VITAMINS:		WATER:	CUPS
TUESDAY				
	PRENATAL VITAMINS:		WATER:	CUPS
WEDNESDAY				
	PRENATAL VITAMINS:		WATER:	CUPS
THURSDAY				
	PRENATAL VITAMINS:		WATER:	CUPS
FRIDAY				
	PRENATAL VITAMINS:		WATER:	CUPS
SATURDAY				
	PRENATAL VITAMINS:		WATER:	CUPS
SUNDAY				
	PRENATAL VITAMINS:		WATER:	CUPS

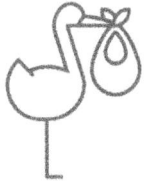

Bump to Baby

week number:

WEIGHT	BELLY SIZE:	DATE

SYMPTOMS:

CRAVINGS AND AVERSIONS:

THOUGHTS AND FEELINGS

BELLY SHOT

NOTES TO BABY:

DEAR BABY,

Meal Planner

week number: [＿＿＿＿＿＿]   TRIMESTER: O FIRST   O SECOND   O THIRD

	BREAKFAST	LUNCH	DINNER	SNACKS
MONDAY				
	PRENATAL VITAMINS:		WATER:	CUPS
TUESDAY				
	PRENATAL VITAMINS:		WATER:	CUPS
WEDNESDAY				
	PRENATAL VITAMINS:		WATER:	CUPS
THURSDAY				
	PRENATAL VITAMINS:		WATER:	CUPS
FRIDAY				
	PRENATAL VITAMINS:		WATER:	CUPS
SATURDAY				
	PRENATAL VITAMINS:		WATER:	CUPS
SUNDAY				
	PRENATAL VITAMINS:		WATER:	CUPS

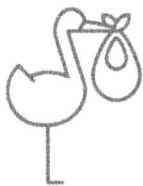

Bump to Baby

week number:

WEIGHT	BELLY SIZE:	DATE

SYMPTOMS:

CRAVINGS AND AVERSIONS:

THOUGHTS AND FEELINGS

BELLY SHOT

NOTES TO BABY:

DEAR BABY,

Meal Planner

week number: [　　　　　　　　]　　TRIMESTER:　O FIRST　O SECOND　O THIRD

	BREAKFAST	LUNCH	DINNER	SNACKS
MONDAY				
	PRENATAL VITAMINS:		WATER:	CUPS
TUESDAY				
	PRENATAL VITAMINS:		WATER:	CUPS
WEDNESDAY				
	PRENATAL VITAMINS:		WATER:	CUPS
THURSDAY				
	PRENATAL VITAMINS:		WATER:	CUPS
FRIDAY				
	PRENATAL VITAMINS:		WATER:	CUPS
SATURDAY				
	PRENATAL VITAMINS:		WATER:	CUPS
SUNDAY				
	PRENATAL VITAMINS:		WATER:	CUPS

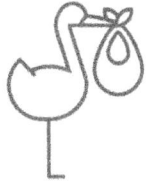

Bump to Baby

week number:

WEIGHT	BELLY SIZE:	DATE

SYMPTOMS:

CRAVINGS AND AVERSIONS:

THOUGHTS AND FEELINGS

BELLY SHOT

NOTES TO BABY:

DEAR BABY,

Meal Planner

week number: [＿＿＿＿＿＿＿]   TRIMESTER: O FIRST   O SECOND   O THIRD

	BREAKFAST	LUNCH	DINNER	SNACKS
MONDAY				
	PRENATAL VITAMINS:		WATER:	CUPS
TUESDAY				
	PRENATAL VITAMINS:		WATER:	CUPS
WEDNESDAY				
	PRENATAL VITAMINS:		WATER:	CUPS
THURSDAY				
	PRENATAL VITAMINS:		WATER:	CUPS
FRIDAY				
	PRENATAL VITAMINS:		WATER:	CUPS
SATURDAY				
	PRENATAL VITAMINS:		WATER:	CUPS
SUNDAY				
	PRENATAL VITAMINS:		WATER:	CUPS

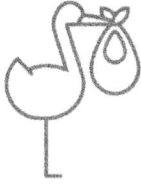

Bump to Baby

week number:

WEIGHT	BELLY SIZE:	DATE

SYMPTOMS:

CRAVINGS AND AVERSIONS:

THOUGHTS AND FEELINGS

BELLY SHOT

NOTES TO BABY:

DEAR BABY,

Meal Planner

week number: [   ]   TRIMESTER: O FIRST   O SECOND   O THIRD

	BREAKFAST	LUNCH	DINNER	SNACKS
MONDAY				
	PRENATAL VITAMINS:		WATER:	CUPS
TUESDAY				
	PRENATAL VITAMINS:		WATER:	CUPS
WEDNESDAY				
	PRENATAL VITAMINS:		WATER:	CUPS
THURSDAY				
	PRENATAL VITAMINS:		WATER:	CUPS
FRIDAY				
	PRENATAL VITAMINS:		WATER:	CUPS
SATURDAY				
	PRENATAL VITAMINS:		WATER:	CUPS
SUNDAY				
	PRENATAL VITAMINS:		WATER:	CUPS

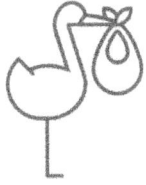

Bump to Baby

week number:

WEIGHT	BELLY SIZE:	DATE

SYMPTOMS:

CRAVINGS AND AVERSIONS:

THOUGHTS AND FEELINGS

BELLY SHOT

NOTES TO BABY:

DEAR BABY,

Meal Planner

week number: [＿＿＿＿＿＿＿]　TRIMESTER:　O FIRST　O SECOND　O THIRD

	BREAKFAST	LUNCH	DINNER	SNACKS
MONDAY				
	PRENATAL VITAMINS:		WATER:	CUPS
TUESDAY				
	PRENATAL VITAMINS:		WATER:	CUPS
WEDNESDAY				
	PRENATAL VITAMINS:		WATER:	CUPS
THURSDAY				
	PRENATAL VITAMINS:		WATER:	CUPS
FRIDAY				
	PRENATAL VITAMINS:		WATER:	CUPS
SATURDAY				
	PRENATAL VITAMINS:		WATER:	CUPS
SUNDAY				
	PRENATAL VITAMINS:		WATER:	CUPS

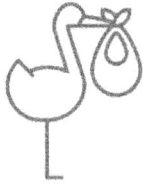

Bump to Baby

week number: [ ]

WEIGHT	BELLY SIZE:	DATE

SYMPTOMS:	CRAVINGS AND AVERSIONS:

THOUGHTS AND FEELINGS	BELLY SHOT

NOTES TO BABY:	
DEAR BABY,	

Meal Planner

week number: [_____]   TRIMESTER: O FIRST   O SECOND   O THIRD

	BREAKFAST	LUNCH	DINNER	SNACKS
MONDAY				
	PRENATAL VITAMINS:		WATER:	CUPS
TUESDAY				
	PRENATAL VITAMINS:		WATER:	CUPS
WEDNESDAY				
	PRENATAL VITAMINS:		WATER:	CUPS
THURSDAY				
	PRENATAL VITAMINS:		WATER:	CUPS
FRIDAY				
	PRENATAL VITAMINS:		WATER:	CUPS
SATURDAY				
	PRENATAL VITAMINS:		WATER:	CUPS
SUNDAY				
	PRENATAL VITAMINS:		WATER:	CUPS

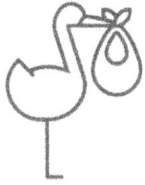

Bump to Baby

week number: [ ]

WEIGHT	BELLY SIZE:	DATE

SYMPTOMS:	CRAVINGS AND AVERSIONS:

THOUGHTS AND FEELINGS	BELLY SHOT

NOTES TO BABY:

DEAR BABY,

Meal Planner

week number: [   ]   TRIMESTER: O FIRST   O SECOND   O THIRD

	BREAKFAST	LUNCH	DINNER	SNACKS
MONDAY				
	PRENATAL VITAMINS:		WATER:	CUPS
TUESDAY				
	PRENATAL VITAMINS:		WATER:	CUPS
WEDNESDAY				
	PRENATAL VITAMINS:		WATER:	CUPS
THURSDAY				
	PRENATAL VITAMINS:		WATER:	CUPS
FRIDAY				
	PRENATAL VITAMINS:		WATER:	CUPS
SATURDAY				
	PRENATAL VITAMINS:		WATER:	CUPS
SUNDAY				
	PRENATAL VITAMINS:		WATER:	CUPS

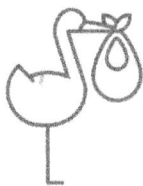

Bump to Baby

week number: [ ]

WEIGHT	BELLY SIZE:	DATE

SYMPTOMS:

CRAVINGS AND AVERSIONS:

THOUGHTS AND FEELINGS

BELLY SHOT

NOTES TO BABY:

DEAR BABY,

Meal Planner

week number: [　　　　　　]   TRIMESTER: O FIRST   O SECOND   O THIRD

	BREAKFAST	LUNCH	DINNER	SNACKS
MONDAY				
	PRENATAL VITAMINS:		WATER:	CUPS
TUESDAY				
	PRENATAL VITAMINS:		WATER:	CUPS
WEDNESDAY				
	PRENATAL VITAMINS:		WATER:	CUPS
THURSDAY				
	PRENATAL VITAMINS:		WATER:	CUPS
FRIDAY				
	PRENATAL VITAMINS:		WATER:	CUPS
SATURDAY				
	PRENATAL VITAMINS:		WATER:	CUPS
SUNDAY				
	PRENATAL VITAMINS:		WATER:	CUPS

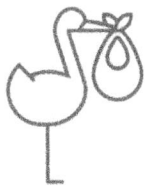

Bump to Baby

week number:

WEIGHT	BELLY SIZE:	DATE

SYMPTOMS:

CRAVINGS AND AVERSIONS:

THOUGHTS AND FEELINGS

BELLY SHOT

NOTES TO BABY:

DEAR BABY,

Meal Planner

week number: [＿＿＿＿＿＿]   TRIMESTER: O FIRST   O SECOND   O THIRD

	BREAKFAST	LUNCH	DINNER	SNACKS
MONDAY				
	PRENATAL VITAMINS:		WATER:	CUPS
TUESDAY				
	PRENATAL VITAMINS:		WATER:	CUPS
WEDNESDAY				
	PRENATAL VITAMINS:		WATER:	CUPS
THURSDAY				
	PRENATAL VITAMINS:		WATER:	CUPS
FRIDAY				
	PRENATAL VITAMINS:		WATER:	CUPS
SATURDAY				
	PRENATAL VITAMINS:		WATER:	CUPS
SUNDAY				
	PRENATAL VITAMINS:		WATER:	CUPS

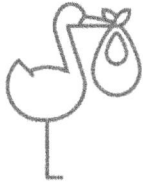

Bump to Baby

week number:

WEIGHT	BELLY SIZE:	DATE

SYMPTOMS:

CRAVINGS AND AVERSIONS:

THOUGHTS AND FEELINGS

BELLY SHOT

NOTES TO BABY:

DEAR BABY,

Meal Planner

week number: [   ]   TRIMESTER: O FIRST   O SECOND   O THIRD

	BREAKFAST	LUNCH	DINNER	SNACKS
MONDAY				
	PRENATAL VITAMINS:		WATER:	CUPS
TUESDAY				
	PRENATAL VITAMINS:		WATER:	CUPS
WEDNESDAY				
	PRENATAL VITAMINS:		WATER:	CUPS
THURSDAY				
	PRENATAL VITAMINS:		WATER:	CUPS
FRIDAY				
	PRENATAL VITAMINS:		WATER:	CUPS
SATURDAY				
	PRENATAL VITAMINS:		WATER:	CUPS
SUNDAY				
	PRENATAL VITAMINS:		WATER:	CUPS

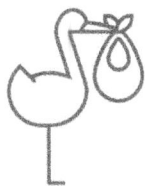

Bump to Baby

week number:

WEIGHT	BELLY SIZE:	DATE

SYMPTOMS:

CRAVINGS AND AVERSIONS:

THOUGHTS AND FEELINGS

BELLY SHOT

NOTES TO BABY:

DEAR BABY,

Meal Planner

week number: [   ]   TRIMESTER: O FIRST   O SECOND   O THIRD

	BREAKFAST	LUNCH	DINNER	SNACKS
MONDAY				
	PRENATAL VITAMINS:		WATER:	CUPS
TUESDAY				
	PRENATAL VITAMINS:		WATER:	CUPS
WEDNESDAY				
	PRENATAL VITAMINS:		WATER:	CUPS
THURSDAY				
	PRENATAL VITAMINS:		WATER:	CUPS
FRIDAY				
	PRENATAL VITAMINS:		WATER:	CUPS
SATURDAY				
	PRENATAL VITAMINS:		WATER:	CUPS
SUNDAY				
	PRENATAL VITAMINS:		WATER:	CUPS

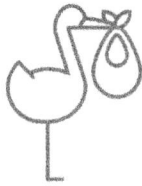

Bump to Baby

week number:

WEIGHT	BELLY SIZE:	DATE

SYMPTOMS:	CRAVINGS AND AVERSIONS:

THOUGHTS AND FEELINGS	BELLY SHOT

NOTES TO BABY:

DEAR BABY,

Meal Planner

week number: [   ]   TRIMESTER: O FIRST   O SECOND   O THIRD

	BREAKFAST	LUNCH	DINNER	SNACKS
MONDAY				
	PRENATAL VITAMINS:		WATER:	CUPS
TUESDAY				
	PRENATAL VITAMINS:		WATER:	CUPS
WEDNESDAY				
	PRENATAL VITAMINS:		WATER:	CUPS
THURSDAY				
	PRENATAL VITAMINS:		WATER:	CUPS
FRIDAY				
	PRENATAL VITAMINS:		WATER:	CUPS
SATURDAY				
	PRENATAL VITAMINS:		WATER:	CUPS
SUNDAY				
	PRENATAL VITAMINS:		WATER:	CUPS

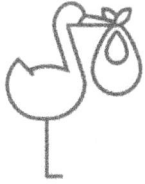

Bump to Baby

week number:

WEIGHT	BELLY SIZE:	DATE

SYMPTOMS:

CRAVINGS AND AVERSIONS:

THOUGHTS AND FEELINGS

BELLY SHOT

NOTES TO BABY:

DEAR BABY,

Meal Planner

week number: [　　　　　　　]　TRIMESTER:　O FIRST　O SECOND　O THIRD

	BREAKFAST	LUNCH	DINNER	SNACKS
MONDAY				
	PRENATAL VITAMINS:		WATER:	CUPS
TUESDAY				
	PRENATAL VITAMINS:		WATER:	CUPS
WEDNESDAY				
	PRENATAL VITAMINS:		WATER:	CUPS
THURSDAY				
	PRENATAL VITAMINS:		WATER:	CUPS
FRIDAY				
	PRENATAL VITAMINS:		WATER:	CUPS
SATURDAY				
	PRENATAL VITAMINS:		WATER:	CUPS
SUNDAY				
	PRENATAL VITAMINS:		WATER:	CUPS

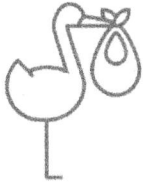

Bump to Baby

week number: [ ]

WEIGHT	BELLY SIZE:	DATE

SYMPTOMS:

CRAVINGS AND AVERSIONS:

THOUGHTS AND FEELINGS

BELLY SHOT

NOTES TO BABY:

DEAR BABY,

Meal Planner

week number: [   ]   TRIMESTER: O FIRST   O SECOND   O THIRD

	BREAKFAST	LUNCH	DINNER	SNACKS
MONDAY				
	PRENATAL VITAMINS:		WATER:	CUPS
TUESDAY				
	PRENATAL VITAMINS:		WATER:	CUPS
WEDNESDAY				
	PRENATAL VITAMINS:		WATER:	CUPS
THURSDAY				
	PRENATAL VITAMINS:		WATER:	CUPS
FRIDAY				
	PRENATAL VITAMINS:		WATER:	CUPS
SATURDAY				
	PRENATAL VITAMINS:		WATER:	CUPS
SUNDAY				
	PRENATAL VITAMINS:		WATER:	CUPS

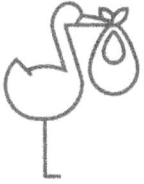

Bump to Baby

week number:

WEIGHT	BELLY SIZE:	DATE

SYMPTOMS:

CRAVINGS AND AVERSIONS:

THOUGHTS AND FEELINGS

BELLY SHOT

NOTES TO BABY:

DEAR BABY,

Meal Planner

week number: [_____] TRIMESTER: O FIRST   O SECOND   O THIRD

	BREAKFAST	LUNCH	DINNER	SNACKS
MONDAY				
	PRENATAL VITAMINS:		WATER:	CUPS
TUESDAY				
	PRENATAL VITAMINS:		WATER:	CUPS
WEDNESDAY				
	PRENATAL VITAMINS:		WATER:	CUPS
THURSDAY				
	PRENATAL VITAMINS:		WATER:	CUPS
FRIDAY				
	PRENATAL VITAMINS:		WATER:	CUPS
SATURDAY				
	PRENATAL VITAMINS:		WATER:	CUPS
SUNDAY				
	PRENATAL VITAMINS:		WATER:	CUPS

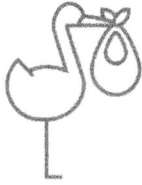

Bump to Baby

week number:

WEIGHT	BELLY SIZE:	DATE

SYMPTOMS:

CRAVINGS AND AVERSIONS:

THOUGHTS AND FEELINGS

BELLY SHOT

NOTES TO BABY:

DEAR BABY,

Meal Planner

week number: [   ]   TRIMESTER: O FIRST   O SECOND   O THIRD

	BREAKFAST	LUNCH	DINNER	SNACKS
MONDAY				
	PRENATAL VITAMINS:		WATER:	CUPS
TUESDAY				
	PRENATAL VITAMINS:		WATER:	CUPS
WEDNESDAY				
	PRENATAL VITAMINS:		WATER:	CUPS
THURSDAY				
	PRENATAL VITAMINS:		WATER:	CUPS
FRIDAY				
	PRENATAL VITAMINS:		WATER:	CUPS
SATURDAY				
	PRENATAL VITAMINS:		WATER:	CUPS
SUNDAY				
	PRENATAL VITAMINS:		WATER:	CUPS

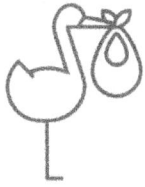

Bump to Baby

week number:

WEIGHT	BELLY SIZE:	DATE

SYMPTOMS:	CRAVINGS AND AVERSIONS:

THOUGHTS AND FEELINGS	BELLY SHOT

NOTES TO BABY:

DEAR BABY,

Meal Planner

week number: [_____]   TRIMESTER: O FIRST   O SECOND   O THIRD

	BREAKFAST	LUNCH	DINNER	SNACKS
MONDAY				
	PRENATAL VITAMINS:		WATER:	CUPS
TUESDAY				
	PRENATAL VITAMINS:		WATER:	CUPS
WEDNESDAY				
	PRENATAL VITAMINS:		WATER:	CUPS
THURSDAY				
	PRENATAL VITAMINS:		WATER:	CUPS
FRIDAY				
	PRENATAL VITAMINS:		WATER:	CUPS
SATURDAY				
	PRENATAL VITAMINS:		WATER:	CUPS
SUNDAY				
	PRENATAL VITAMINS:		WATER:	CUPS

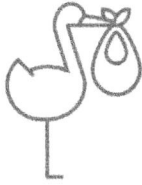

Bump to Baby

week number:

WEIGHT	BELLY SIZE:	DATE

SYMPTOMS:

CRAVINGS AND AVERSIONS:

THOUGHTS AND FEELINGS

BELLY SHOT

NOTES TO BABY:

DEAR BABY,

Meal Planner

week number: [_____] TRIMESTER: O FIRST O SECOND O THIRD

	BREAKFAST	LUNCH	DINNER	SNACKS
MONDAY				
	PRENATAL VITAMINS:		WATER:	CUPS
TUESDAY				
	PRENATAL VITAMINS:		WATER:	CUPS
WEDNESDAY				
	PRENATAL VITAMINS:		WATER:	CUPS
THURSDAY				
	PRENATAL VITAMINS:		WATER:	CUPS
FRIDAY				
	PRENATAL VITAMINS:		WATER:	CUPS
SATURDAY				
	PRENATAL VITAMINS:		WATER:	CUPS
SUNDAY				
	PRENATAL VITAMINS:		WATER:	CUPS

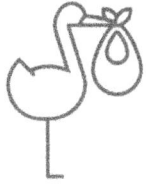

Bump to Baby

week number:

WEIGHT	BELLY SIZE:	DATE

SYMPTOMS:	CRAVINGS AND AVERSIONS:

THOUGHTS AND FEELINGS	BELLY SHOT

NOTES TO BABY:

DEAR BABY,

Meal Planner

week number: [_____]   TRIMESTER: O FIRST   O SECOND   O THIRD

	BREAKFAST	LUNCH	DINNER	SNACKS
MONDAY				
	PRENATAL VITAMINS:		WATER:	CUPS
TUESDAY				
	PRENATAL VITAMINS:		WATER:	CUPS
WEDNESDAY				
	PRENATAL VITAMINS:		WATER:	CUPS
THURSDAY				
	PRENATAL VITAMINS:		WATER:	CUPS
FRIDAY				
	PRENATAL VITAMINS:		WATER:	CUPS
SATURDAY				
	PRENATAL VITAMINS:		WATER:	CUPS
SUNDAY				
	PRENATAL VITAMINS:		WATER:	CUPS

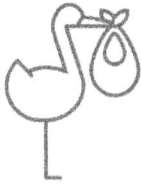

Bump to Baby

week number:

WEIGHT	BELLY SIZE:	DATE

SYMPTOMS:

CRAVINGS AND AVERSIONS:

THOUGHTS AND FEELINGS

BELLY SHOT

NOTES TO BABY:

DEAR BABY,

Meal Planner

week number: [   ]   TRIMESTER: O FIRST   O SECOND   O THIRD

	BREAKFAST	LUNCH	DINNER	SNACKS
MONDAY				
	PRENATAL VITAMINS:		WATER:	CUPS
TUESDAY				
	PRENATAL VITAMINS:		WATER:	CUPS
WEDNESDAY				
	PRENATAL VITAMINS:		WATER:	CUPS
THURSDAY				
	PRENATAL VITAMINS:		WATER:	CUPS
FRIDAY				
	PRENATAL VITAMINS:		WATER:	CUPS
SATURDAY				
	PRENATAL VITAMINS:		WATER:	CUPS
SUNDAY				
	PRENATAL VITAMINS:		WATER:	CUPS

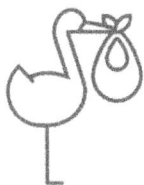

Bump to Baby

week number: [ ]

WEIGHT	BELLY SIZE:	DATE

SYMPTOMS:	CRAVINGS AND AVERSIONS:

THOUGHTS AND FEELINGS	BELLY SHOT

NOTES TO BABY:
DEAR BABY,

Meal Planner

week number: [   ]   TRIMESTER: O FIRST   O SECOND   O THIRD

	BREAKFAST	LUNCH	DINNER	SNACKS
MONDAY				
	PRENATAL VITAMINS:		WATER:	CUPS
TUESDAY				
	PRENATAL VITAMINS:		WATER:	CUPS
WEDNESDAY				
	PRENATAL VITAMINS:		WATER:	CUPS
THURSDAY				
	PRENATAL VITAMINS:		WATER:	CUPS
FRIDAY				
	PRENATAL VITAMINS:		WATER:	CUPS
SATURDAY				
	PRENATAL VITAMINS:		WATER:	CUPS
SUNDAY				
	PRENATAL VITAMINS:		WATER:	CUPS

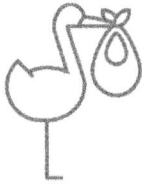

Bump to Baby

week number:

WEIGHT	BELLY SIZE:	DATE

SYMPTOMS:	CRAVINGS AND AVERSIONS:

THOUGHTS AND FEELINGS	BELLY SHOT

NOTES TO BABY:

DEAR BABY,

Meal Planner

week number: [　　　　　　　]　　TRIMESTER: O FIRST　O SECOND　　O THIRD

	BREAKFAST	LUNCH	DINNER	SNACKS
MONDAY				
	PRENATAL VITAMINS:		WATER:	CUPS
TUESDAY				
	PRENATAL VITAMINS:		WATER:	CUPS
WEDNESDAY				
	PRENATAL VITAMINS:		WATER:	CUPS
THURSDAY				
	PRENATAL VITAMINS:		WATER:	CUPS
FRIDAY				
	PRENATAL VITAMINS:		WATER:	CUPS
SATURDAY				
	PRENATAL VITAMINS:		WATER:	CUPS
SUNDAY				
	PRENATAL VITAMINS:		WATER:	CUPS

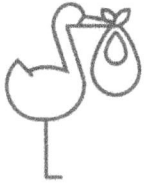

Bump to Baby

week number:

WEIGHT	BELLY SIZE:	DATE

SYMPTOMS:

CRAVINGS AND AVERSIONS:

THOUGHTS AND FEELINGS

BELLY SHOT

NOTES TO BABY:

DEAR BABY,

Meal Planner

week number: [   ]   TRIMESTER: O FIRST   O SECOND   O THIRD

	BREAKFAST	LUNCH	DINNER	SNACKS
MONDAY				
	PRENATAL VITAMINS:		WATER:	CUPS
TUESDAY				
	PRENATAL VITAMINS:		WATER:	CUPS
WEDNESDAY				
	PRENATAL VITAMINS:		WATER:	CUPS
THURSDAY				
	PRENATAL VITAMINS:		WATER:	CUPS
FRIDAY				
	PRENATAL VITAMINS:		WATER:	CUPS
SATURDAY				
	PRENATAL VITAMINS:		WATER:	CUPS
SUNDAY				
	PRENATAL VITAMINS:		WATER:	CUPS

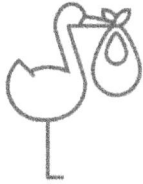

Bump to Baby

week number:

WEIGHT	BELLY SIZE:	DATE

SYMPTOMS:	CRAVINGS AND AVERSIONS:

THOUGHTS AND FEELINGS	BELLY SHOT

NOTES TO BABY:

DEAR BABY,

Meal Planner

week number: [   ]   TRIMESTER: O FIRST   O SECOND   O THIRD

	BREAKFAST	LUNCH	DINNER	SNACKS
MONDAY				
	PRENATAL VITAMINS:		WATER:	CUPS
TUESDAY				
	PRENATAL VITAMINS:		WATER:	CUPS
WEDNESDAY				
	PRENATAL VITAMINS:		WATER:	CUPS
THURSDAY				
	PRENATAL VITAMINS:		WATER:	CUPS
FRIDAY				
	PRENATAL VITAMINS:		WATER:	CUPS
SATURDAY				
	PRENATAL VITAMINS:		WATER:	CUPS
SUNDAY				
	PRENATAL VITAMINS:		WATER:	CUPS

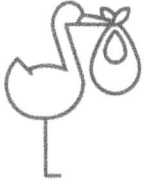

Bump to Baby

week number:

WEIGHT	BELLY SIZE:	DATE

SYMPTOMS:

CRAVINGS AND AVERSIONS:

THOUGHTS AND FEELINGS

BELLY SHOT

NOTES TO BABY:

DEAR BABY,

Meal Planner

week number: [＿＿＿＿＿＿]   TRIMESTER: O FIRST   O SECOND   O THIRD

	BREAKFAST	LUNCH	DINNER	SNACKS
MONDAY				
	PRENATAL VITAMINS:		WATER:	CUPS
TUESDAY				
	PRENATAL VITAMINS:		WATER:	CUPS
WEDNESDAY				
	PRENATAL VITAMINS:		WATER:	CUPS
THURSDAY				
	PRENATAL VITAMINS:		WATER:	CUPS
FRIDAY				
	PRENATAL VITAMINS:		WATER:	CUPS
SATURDAY				
	PRENATAL VITAMINS:		WATER:	CUPS
SUNDAY				
	PRENATAL VITAMINS:		WATER:	CUPS

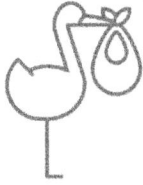

Bump to Baby

week number:

WEIGHT	BELLY SIZE:	DATE

SYMPTOMS:

CRAVINGS AND AVERSIONS:

THOUGHTS AND FEELINGS

BELLY SHOT

NOTES TO BABY:

DEAR BABY,

www.ingramcontent.com/pod-product-compliance
Lightning Source LLC
Chambersburg PA
CBHW081148020426
42333CB00021B/2701